THE LITTLE BOOK OF HEALTH & WEIGHT LOSS

BY VALENCIA DANTZLER

Introduction:

The purpose of this book is to outline the four steps to better health and weight loss that I have adopted. This is the actual route that I took to transform my life to lose weight; to feel better; and to look younger. I feel better than I've ever felt in all my life. It is my purpose and my duty to bring these steps to you and to let you know that you can start from wherever you are right now. Let go of the past. The past does not matter! What matters is standing where you are right now and moving forward in the direction in which you want to go! The secret, if there is a secret, is to keep your eye on where you want to be and every day to take steps to go in that direction. I'm a Living Testament that you can do it, that you can get there from where you are TODAY!

My Story:

For almost 50 years I struggled with the issues of being unhealthy and overweight. I saw my mother die of diabetes, My grandfather died of a heart attack before he was 55, my grandmother died of breast cancer, and high blood pressure ran through my family history. Growing up I was the fattest kid on the Block, and I got called all the names you could think of. Later in 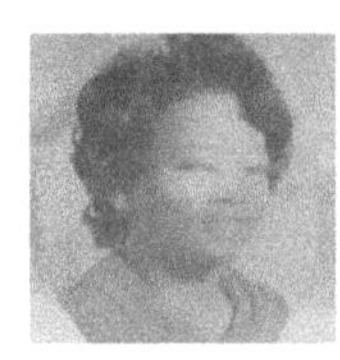 my life, I continued my struggle with health and weight loss issues. I saw my mother die from complications of diabetes by the time I was seven years old. So, I decided to dedicate my service to the community in her honor by serving as an EMT with the local ambulance company.   For six years, I saved lives and tended to the sick. While I was there, I saw so many people who were down and out on their luck.   I tended to all walks of life, from The Homeless to The Millionaires living in Mansions, who wanted to commit suicide. I had my "regulars" who began to be not so sick, but as they took their prescription medications that the doctor prescribed for them, I saw them get sicker and sicker as time went on.   Growing up in the church, I prayed to God.   I said, "God I see my people getting sicker and sicker taking these medications, but I don't see them getting any better for the most part." I got a chance to talk with several prominent doctors, and surgeons, and ask them questions. I asked the doctors how much education did they get in there 8 to 10 years of study on Natural Medicine. I was surprised when one prominent doctor told me, "Oh…. about two weeks"!! I was shocked when he told me that. But then it all started to make sense. Now I knew that the whole industry makes money as long as people are sick.   Imagine if the world was mostly healthy, hospitals, pharmaceutical & insurance companies would go bankrupt!

I was on medication for High Blood Pressure and was always tired and irritable. These medications are not natural. They are synthetic. Is our body designed to accept and assimilate things that are unnatural totally?   I asked God, "If you made us, then don't you have something natural for us"?   And with that one question, my quest for better health for myself and my World…... BEGAN!

My quest has led me to a younger appearance, more energy, a sustained weight loss of over 60 lbs to date, and more Vitality than ever before and….. yes I'm off all medications at the age of 50!

How did I do it, I used my 4 Steps to Health & Weight Loss…...

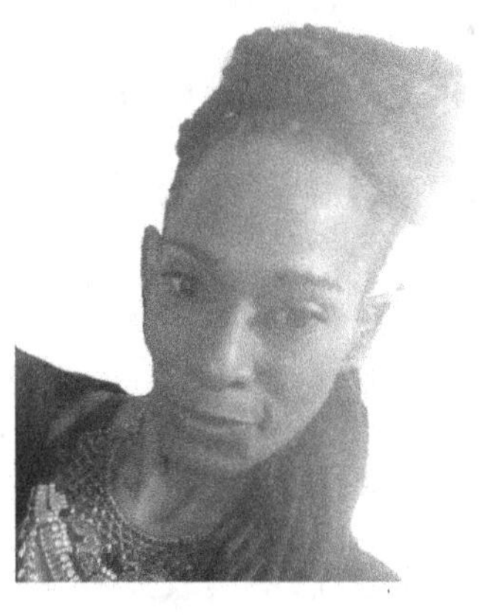

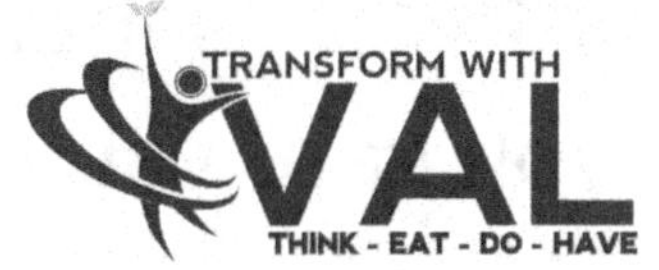

4 Steps to Health & Weight Loss:
What You **Think**
What You **Eat**
What You **Do**

What You **Have**

Step 1: What You Think

Decision:

There's an old adage that says, " what you think about you bring about" and "you are what you think." This is true in all walks of life, and your health should be no different. If you think you can, you can. If you think you MUST, don't worry you WILL! If you have gotten to a point where enough is enough…….. Excellent! Now you're ready to begin your journey because there's no giving up there is NO GIVING IN! Should you fall, as long as you can look up, you can get up …..Remember that! The hardest part of this journey is to get your mind right. There's going to be times when you don't feel like it. There's going to be times when you feel like you simply cannot do it. But I want you to know that this is normal and to expect it. Take Authority, in spite of how you feel; you're going to take it one hour and one day at a time.   I want you to DECIDE right NOW to take authority over your body Knowing that you have complete control over all areas of your life. Mindset is everything!

Goals & Pictures:
  The first thing you're going to have to do it set a goal and write it down. Then, I don't want you just to write it down. Now, you must picture it. Go through some

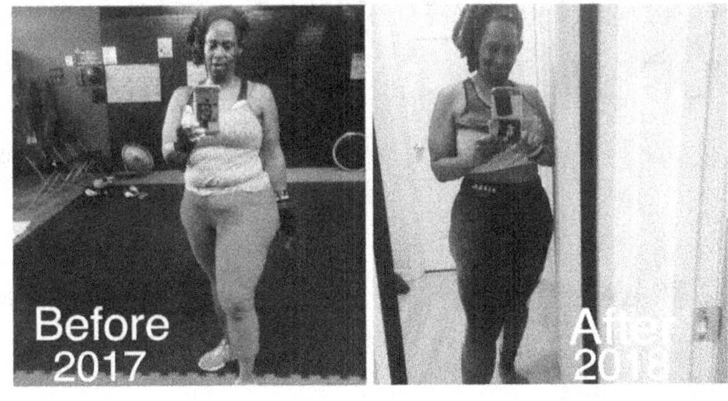

magazines, go online & save some pictures on your phone to get a picture of what you want and get them printed out. If it's a certain body type, then cut the head off and paste a picture of your head onto that body and put it on your wall so that you can see it every day. Look at it each day. Put it on the light switch in your bedroom, at least you'll see it twice a day. You don't even have to look at it directly but it's there, and your subconscious mind is picking it up, and you are becoming that picture on your wall. So, when you get to the point to where you are working out. You're going to remember that picture, and it's going to be just what you need to take you over the edge and get through that moment. Just remember, you get what you PICTURE in life, not what you want!

Step 2: What You Eat

Small choices lead to BIG Changes!

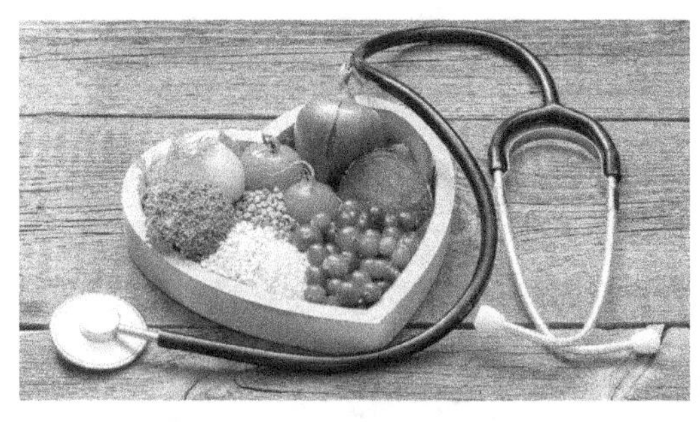

Imhotep originally said "Let food be thy medicine and medicine be thy food," but it doesn't mean it has to be nasty in taste!! You've got to know that you are already most likely going to associate fat, salt and sugar as tasting wonderful. And to be honest, it does! But, you have to know that there are good, better and best choices that you can make. In a nutshell, you're going to have to increase your vegetable intake. In fact, the more veggies you eat, the better! The higher quality of vegetables, The BEST! The more Alkaline your food, the healthier you will be. I pretty much throw calories out the window and concentrate on eating the most nutritious foods I can find. My daily goal is to

ELIMINATE as many processed foods as I can. When in doubt, stick with the natural state of foods as close to the way that God has made them.

Cleansing your insides is just as important as cleansing your skin and outer body. Your body must be cleansed of parasites and toxins that seem to control it.   Toxins and chemicals seep in from the air that we breathe, the food that we eat, the water that we drink, and even down to the lotions, perfumes, and potions that we put on our skin. As our inner body is cleansed, the body tends to relax because it is no longer in the State of Emergency. In other words, it tends to relax and not try to hold on to fat to protect the vital organs that are found in the midsection,(i.e., stomach area). Weight and inches are then released, and we start to feel better and even have more energy and clarity of thought. Eating a majority of

Alkaline Foods is a way of cleansing and detoxing the body on a regular basis. This is what Hippocrates meant by "Food being thy medicine." Disease is much more attracted to an Acidic state and truly cannot exist in a more Alkaline Body. So what makes the body Acidic? Meats, Starchy foods, and Sugar just to name a few. However, Alkalinity is very high in green, leafy vegetables. In fact, the more green vegetables you eat, the healthier and leaner you will tend to be. Now, I'm not saying only eat green. Just know that the greener a vegetable and the less starch that you eat, the healthier you will be.

Good, Better, BEST Food Chart:

Vegetables

Good	Better	BEST
Store Bought	Locally Grown	Organic
	Zucchini, squash	
Potatoes	Red Potatoes	Organic Red Potatoes
Broccoli, Cauliflower, Carrots	Beans, Lentils	Chickpeas (Garbanzo Beans)
String Beans	Greens: Collards, Kale, Romaine Lettuce	Any Organic Green Leafy Vegetable
	Collard Greens	
	Spinach	Greens, Kale, All lettuce (Except Iceberg), Turnip Greens, Okra, Olives, Onions, Green Banana
		Sea Vegetables
		Squash, Zucchini
		Cherry & Plum Tomatoes
		Mushrooms (Except Shitake)
		Avocado (No Seedless)

		Bell Peppers
		Cucumbers

Fruits

Good	Better	BEST
	Fruit with the Seed!	Organic
	Grape or Plum Tomatoes	Avocado (No Seedless)
	Hard Coconuts	Apples, Cherries Small Bananas Burro Bananas All Berries (No Cranberries) Currants, Dates, Figs, Grapes (Seeded), Limes, Mango, Seeded Melons, Papaya, Peach, Pear, Plums, Raisins (Seeded), Soft Jelly Coconut, Soursop, Tamarind

Dairy, Nuts & Seeds

good	Better	BEST
Soy Milk	Almond Milk, Almond Butter	Coconut Milk Brazil Nut Milk

Organic Milk (Cow), Peanuts, Peanut Butter	Pecans, Macadamia Nuts, Cashews	Hemp seeds, Tahini, Walnuts, Brazil Nuts

Meats

good	Better	BEST
		No Meat
	Organic Poultry & Eggs	
Fresh Fish	Wild-Caught Salmon	

Fats, Sugars & Salts

good	Better	BEST
	Brown Sugar, Erythritol	Agave, Stevia, Coconut Sugar, Monk Fruit Sugar
Olive Oil	Virgin Olive Oil, Coconut Oil	Grapeseed Oil (For Cooking)
	Non-Iodized Salt	Sea Salt, Himalayan Salt
	Bragg's Aminos	Coconut Oil (Do Not Cook)
		Sesame Oil, Hemp seed Oil, Avocado Oil

Grains, Bread & Pastas

Good	Better	Best
Whole Grain	Bean, Lentil	Chickpea (Garbanzo), Spelt
Brown Rice	Wild Rice	Amaranth, Fonio, Kamut
		Quinoa, Rye, Teff

Step 3: What You Do

There's a philosophy that I have come to know to be very true. As you feel better, you're going to do better.   So, give yourself at least 30 Minutes of Love each day. Love is my Code Name for exercise. Even if it's just walking, you deserve to Love Yourself. Remember if you don't Love Yourself, nobody else will either! I must say, that it took me a very long time to learn to love exercise. In fact, I would never put those two words together: Love & Exercise. But, as I learned to eat more healthy, and gently cleanse my blood and organs, I began to feel much better, and my energy increased. With increased energy, my outlook on life became much better, and I wanted to be more active. I began to give myself the gift of 30 minutes of Love each day. I decided that I was worth at least 30 minutes. So, I began to walk around in my neighborhood and spend time with God observing the Nature that He has given us. It became a deep and spiritual practice for me, and I began to look forward to it each day. That was my time with Him!

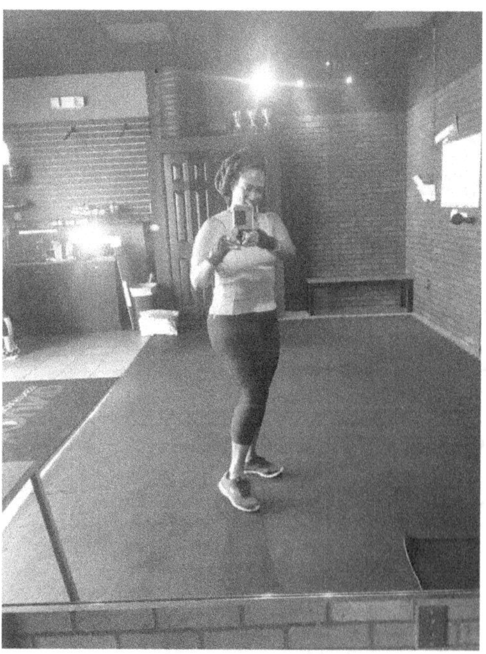

So, right now, I want you to DECIDE when you are going to give yourself 30 Minutes of Love. You've got to be consistent. So, put it on your calendar right now for each day of the week (at least 5 days a week). You may start out just walking or going to the gym during the week. Perhaps you'd like to change it up on the weekends, and as a family, you and your household can go to the park and play games or go bowling. I mean you do make plans to go out to eat on the weekends, don't you? Well, I think you can plan to get some fun physical activity in as well. Who knows, it may even bring you all even closer together as a family!

Exercise has been known to decrease stress. As we live our lives, stress can tend to bombard us. Stress also can make us fat! So, make it a practice to use your 30 minutes wisely. If you've got a problem or frustration, work it out as you exercise. Use it to your advantage, work it out physically by moving that body and breaking a sweat, and then leave it there! Reduce and then

ELIMINATE that stress, consistently with 30 minutes a day.

Step 4: What You Have

For years, I never realized the impact that supplements can have on your body for speeding up results that you wish to see. In fact, I never even believed in them. I would purchase countless bottles of vitamin pills hoping to get healthy but, it always eluded me.   I never felt I was getting the results that I wanted until I tried a little pack of tea. That little pack of tea changed my life! The tea was from a company called Total Life Changes and is called IASO Tea. During my 1st week on the tea, I lost 6 lbs in 6 days. Coupled with 2 other products, the NutraBurst and the Chaga, the doctor took me off of all medicines within 6 weeks. Now, I'm not here to offer any Medical Claims or to mitigate any diseases. I cannot say that these supplements will cure you.

But, I can give you the benefits of how a few key products work. As far as I'm concerned, they are "Must Haves" for my daily regimine.

Iaso Tea - is mainly a gentle cleanser that you can drink on a daily basis 2 times per day. It cleans the blood and organs on a cellular level as well as rids the body of parasites and sludge that builds up in the intestines over several years.

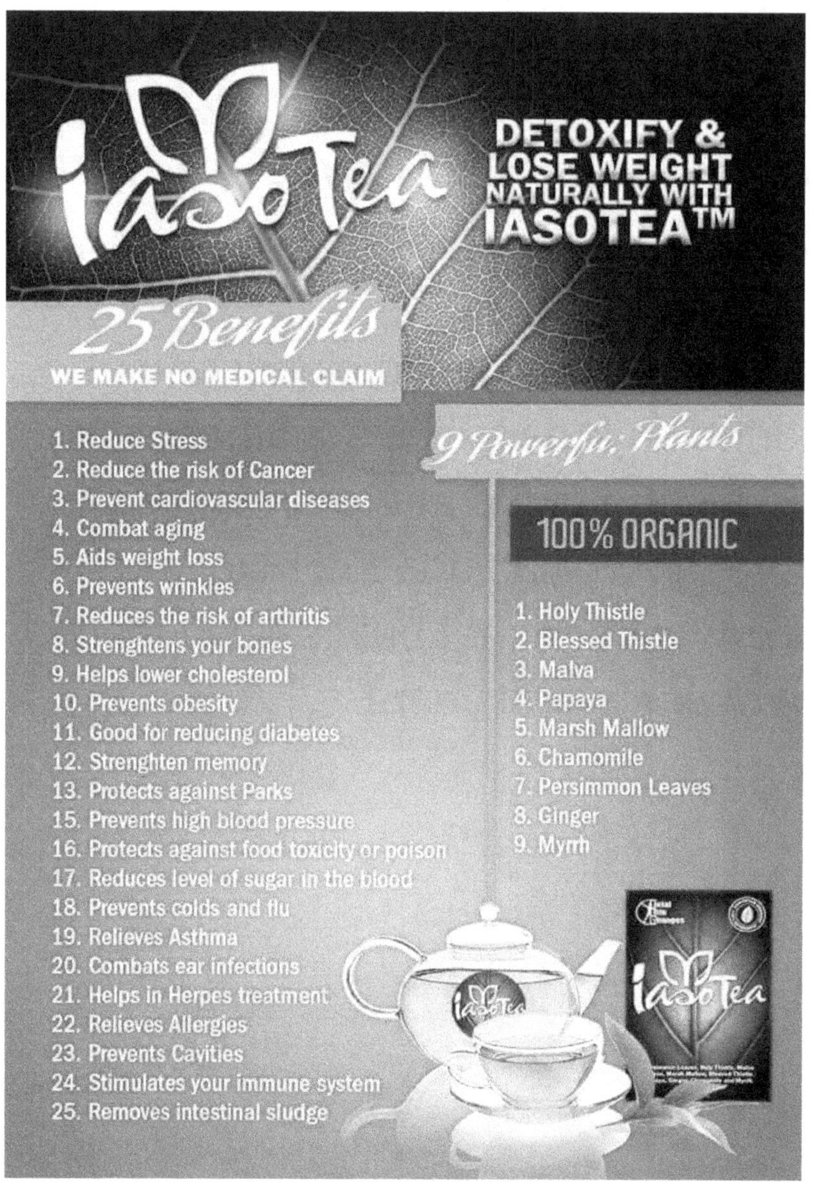

NutraBurst - is a liquid multivitamin and mineral which contains 72 minerals. It builds the body up and rids the body of inflammation which can cause pain. Most of the common vegetables that we eat today are actually hybrids and lack the minerals that our body needs. When the food lacks the essential minerals that our body needs, it pulls what it needs from our bones. Over time, this weakens our bones and ads stress to our body, and we begin to break down. NutraBurst combats this process because it has 72 essential minerals that the body needs. Along with Techui, which consists of salt water spirulina, we have the remaining essential minerals that our body needs to survive.

NRG - is an all natural supplement that gives the body complete energy without jitters or crashing. It also suppresses appetite and causes the body to burn an extra 300 calories per capsule. NRG has also been known to increase concentration

in children and adults all while enhancing
mood with a feeling of happiness.

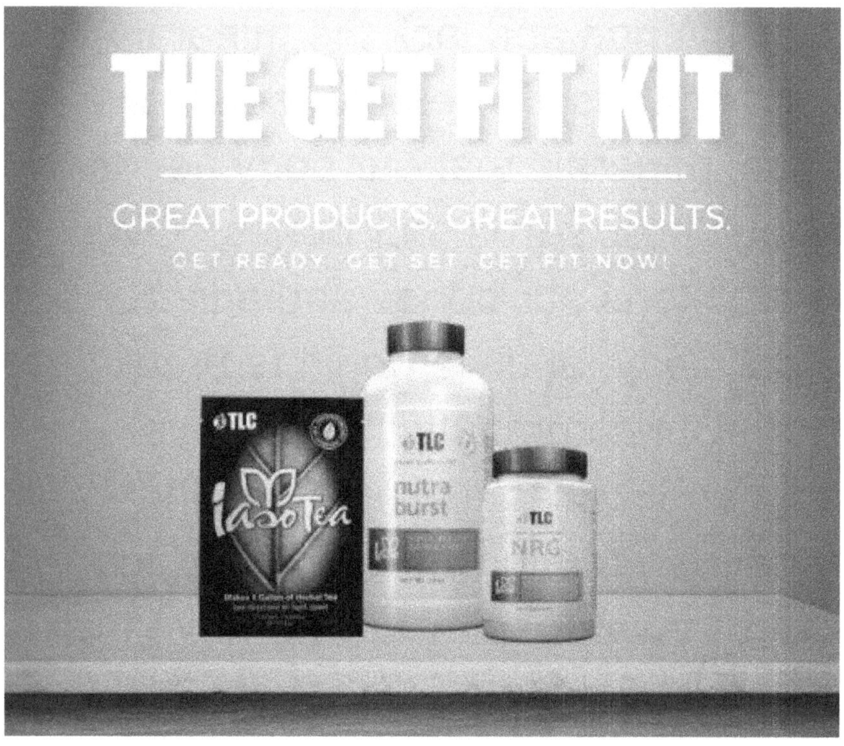

Resolution Drops - The Amazing Resolution
Drops are phenomenal when it comes to
weight loss. They cause most people to lose
1 to 3 pounds a day. While on the Drops,
you must adhere to a strict eating plan of
1200 calories per day which consists mostly
of vegetables, some fruits, and protein. The
Drops is considered your "Coach in a Bottle"

because it sends warning signals to your brain should you go off course. You may have a feeling of sickness or a bad taste should you eat something outside of the eating plan.

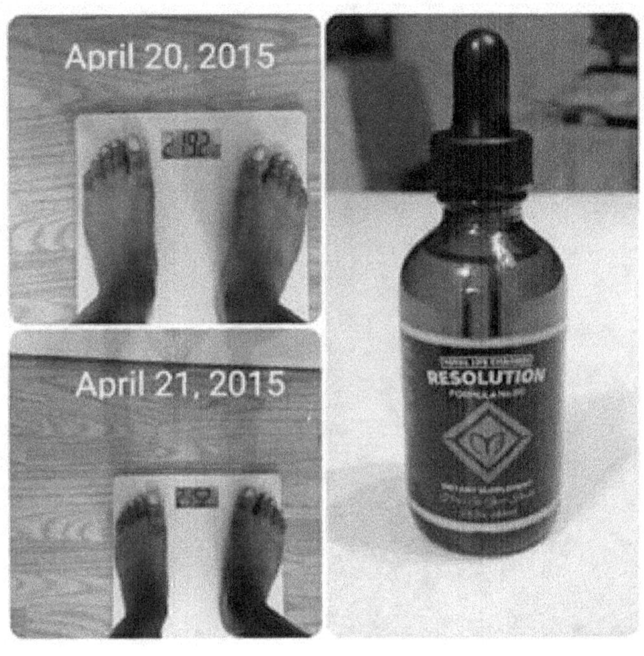

Chaga - is a Medicinal Mushroom that has been around for thousands of years in Chinese Medicine. It is known as God's Gift and grows high up on a tree. Chaga actually travels in the body and seeking and destroying toxins in the body. It detoxes your body on a very high level. It's even been known to eat tumors and has the highest oracle level of any substance known to man. It truly lives up to its name, God's Gift.

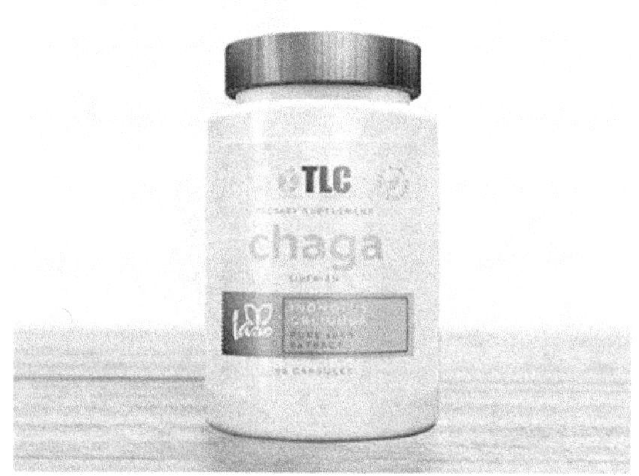

Conclusion:

When you implement these 4 simple steps, I can promise you a few things:

1) It will be harder than you think….at first.
2) It will be easier than you think….ongoing.

3) You will achieve way more than you imagined possible in all areas of your life.

I hope this little booklet has been a blessing to you! There are so many ideas out there for weight loss and better health that it can all be so confusing and complicated. I hope that this booklet keeps it simple for you. Keep this booklet with you as you go through your journey and may it keep you on the path to Health & Wellness. Keep this little booklet in your possession until you reach your Health & Fitness Goal ---and when you do, make me the first person you contact.

God Bless!

Your friend,
Valencia J. Dantzler

TransformWithVal.com
ShopWithValToday.com

For Booking Events, contact 980-613-7301